Life at the Receiving End: The Experiences and Views of an NHS Patient

Pharmacists, Doctors and other Primary Care Services

By

PharmaPatient

Dedication

To my partner who encouraged me to stop complaining

and to write about my experiences and views; to all fellow

patients and to the health professionals whose job it is to

look after our health

Table of Contents

Contents

Prologue

The NHS is a wonderful institution. It was established in 1948 to provide universal access to good quality healthcare for all citizens of the United Kingdom. More often than not it does this very well. It's a shame that we prefer to highlight those times when it doesn't.

I am fortunate to have been born after 1948. Sometimes I take the NHS for granted. I forget what a privilege it is to have this level of care without paying at the point of provision – well – other than when I have to pay the prescription charge at the pharmacy or when I visit an NHS dentist. There are lots of countries, some of them as developed as our own, in which access to good-quality healthcare depends on having personal health insurance or the ability to pay directly for the privilege.

At times I feel that those providing health services take me, as a patient, for granted. It feels like they are just in it "for the money". I am just another statistic – a means to an end. No single group of health professionals stands out when it comes to sub-standard care. I suppose health

i

professionals are a reflection of society in that sense: you get the bad with the good. I think I just expect a higher standard of moral and ethical probity from health professionals due to the power they wield over our lives.

This book outlines some of my experiences and thoughts as a patient using the NHS. I am aware of several books written by health professionals for each other or to "educate" patients on how difficult the lives of health professionals are. However, there are not as many books written by patients for the health professionals. I hope this one helps start a healthy conversation with health professionals in primary care; the people that first attend to us before we are referred to hospital for more invasive procedures.

I wish to thank the anonymous pharmacists and doctors that agreed to proof-read the text before publication. I asked them to check the accuracy of the statements about the inside workings of pharmacy and GP surgeries. I retain accountability for any errors that remain and, indeed, for any errors in the work.

A few of the thoughts in this book are on my website at http://www.pharmapatient.com. Please visit the blog and tell me what you think about this book or any other ideas. You can also follow me on Twitter. Look for @pharmapatient.

Section 1: The Pharmacy

"The work of a pharmacy professional can take many forms and you may work in different settings, including clinical practice, education, research and industry. … The care, well-being and safety of patients are at the heart of professional practice. They must always be your first concern. Even if you do not have direct contact with patients your decisions or behaviour can still affect their care or safety." Standards of Conduct, Ethics and Professional Practice; General Pharmaceutical Council, September 2010.

Accessed January 2013. Hyperlink: http://www.pharmacyregulation.org/sites/default/files/Standards%20of%20conduct,%20ethics%20and%20performance.pdf

1

I love my local pharmacy

Some of the things that you will read in this book will make you think that I am out to "get" pharmacists. This could not be further from the truth. I love my pharmacist and pharmacy in general. I am aware that I owe my very existence to the hard work that pharmacists put in every day of the year. I have seen them save lives and go out of their way to make mine and a lot of customers' lives better.

I recall incidents like the experience of one of my neighbours. Mr Smith (not his real name of course) had gone to the pharmacy to request something over the counter for what he thought was a minor problem. He had been watching television and seen an advertisement for a new treatment for an enlarged prostate in men above a certain age. He felt that he had all the symptoms and thought that the tablets might be just what he needed. The pharmacist spent a few minutes asking Mr Smith some questions and then advised him against buying the tablets; referring him instead to the doctor for an urgent appointment.

The doctor in turn referred him to the local hospital where it was discovered that Mr Smith had prostate cancer. This was a few years ago and Mr Smith is still alive today. He credits the pharmacist with saving his life. I agree with Mr Smith.

I am sure that there are thousands of similar stories up and down the country every day. According to the Health and Social Care Information Centre there were about eleven and a half thousand community pharmacies in England alone by the end of 2013. Each of them dispensed an average of six thousand six hundred items per month. That is a lot of hard work. Finding time to talk to patients and identify potentially life-threatening conditions such as Mr Smith's must call for great skill.

It's not just such stories and the (usually) efficient dispensing that inspire admiration of pharmacists; it's also the other things that pharmacists do that we take for granted. For instance, I have an elderly grandmother whose pharmacy and doctor are located about a mile from where she lives. My grandmother is on a lot of medication and she would be hopelessly confused about how to take them all if she were left to her own resources.

The pharmacy has taken care of her worries (and ours) by managing the reordering of her medication and agreeing to put her medication in blister packs. Her tablets come all neatly laid out by time of day and day of the week in the blister packs. The pharmacy delivers both ad hoc prescriptions when necessary and her regular medication every twenty eight days without fail.

The best part about this is that they do not charge for these services: the deliveries, the reordering and the blister packs are all free. I do not understand the economics behind this. When I order goods online from other retailers there is usually a minimum order value before I can get a free delivery. This does not seem to be the case for pharmacy. I have come to the view that pharmacy must either be so profitable that it can easily absorb the costs; or that the funding model under which pharmacy operates has a provision for such costs.

You would expect that these and many other great things that pharmacists do would mean that we patients are too grateful to complain about the service we get from them. This is sadly not the case. I have seen too many argumentative, upset and angry customers shouting at pharmacists and their staff to be blind to the fact that our emotions as customers can get the better of us at times.

There have been occasions when I have seen people walk up to the counter and ask for their "repeat prescription." The helpful assistants usually ask politely for the customer's name and then check the completed prescriptions to see if one for the patient has been done. If this proves fruitless they check the computer, before turning the pharmacy upside down, to see if a prescription for the patient has been received from the relevant surgery and mislaid in the pharmacy. Often this is not the case. Finally the pharmacist or an unfortunate member of staff does back to the patient and says, almost apologetically,

"We haven't received your prescription from your surgery, Mrs Jones. Are you sure you asked them to send it to us?"

"What do you mean, "ask them to send" it to you?" is a common response. "I told my doctor last time that I use this chemist."

"But did you order the prescription and ask the surgery to put it in our pile for collection?" the member of staff asks.

"Why should I order the prescription again? It should be here. My doctor said it was on repeat. I don't have to go back to see the doctor for another six months. Why haven't you got it?" the patient responds in increasingly agitated tones.

This is usually followed by the pharmacy assistant or the pharmacist explaining what is meant by "repeat prescriptions" and the obligation resting on the patient to reorder the medication on a regular basis unless she has signed up to one of various managed repeat arrangements with either the pharmacy or surgery. On good days the outcome is positive for both the patient and the pharmacy: the pharmacy manages to organise a prescription with the surgery for the patient to collect medication after a day or two. On bad days the patient matches out before hearing the full explanation; at the same time blaming the pharmacy for its "incompetence" and threatening never to return.

I suppose this shows that pharmacy patients are no different to other customers that visit retail outlets. We have a sense of entitlement that sometimes defies logic. We believe that "the customer is always right" and we know that more often than not we will get our way. We know that pharmacies do not want us to complain to anyone outside the pharmacy because they do not want to deal with the potential harm this could cause to their reputations.

The media, for instance, is more likely to be sympathetic to a customer (say a single mum with a young child) than to a branch of a large chain of pharmacies. I remember reading in one of the tabloids a few years ago a story about a pharmacist that had tried to chide a misbehaving child in a branch of one of the big chains. The pharmacist was presented as a monster and the account referred to her as a shop "assistant". While I do not condone the actions that she is alleged to have taken, I found the language in the article deliberately provocative and designed to cast the pharmacist in the worst possible light. Most businesses in today's trading environment know that they cannot easily win a war with the media and they therefore avoid any situations that might bring unwelcome attention. They prefer to relate to the media on their own terms, not the media's.

It is not only the media that pharmacies would rather avoid. As patients we know that pharmacists do not want us to complain to their bosses, the NHS or even the doctor because they do not like the idea of an investigation. The authorities tend to err on the side of the aggrieved patient.

I admit some of my fellow patients play on this to get an unfair advantage over the pharmacist. They abuse refund guarantees or any of a number of things in which there are loopholes. Sadly there's not really much that pharmacists can do about this. Some can b successfully challenged and/or minimised. The rest has to be accepted as the hazard of operating in the service industry.

My highlighting of the abuses above is not intended as a way to justify them. On the contrary it is intended to highlight how; in contrast, most pharmacies provide a smashing service. In the following chapters, any criticisms are presented with the best intentions of forging a better way forward for both patients and pharmacists. In fact, at the end of the pharmacy section I make a few suggestions that pharmacists, in particular, should be very interested in.

The Pharmacy Identity Crisis

Most pharmacists I know work in regular pharmacies on the high street. They sell medicines, perfumes, baby milks, nappies, nicotine replacement products, electronic cigarettes, photography services and, in the bigger shops, clothes and electrical items. I have, in the past, also known pharmacists to sell home brew. They are, without a doubt, storekeepers in every sense of the word.

At the same time they take in our prescriptions from the doctor and give us the items ordered for our illnesses. Once in a while the pharmacist will even ask to talk to me "about my regular medicines" for the cost of my signature (more about this in a later chapter). It seems evident that pharmacists know a lot about drugs and medicines, how to prescribe them as well as how to advise patients on their safe storage and use. They are in this sense highly qualified professionals.

That is where the irony for me lies: How can a storekeeper be a serious health professional at the same time? Imagine, for example, walking into your local GP surgery to find the doctor selling sandwiches and soft drinks, then going to the back and getting the same doctor to examine what could be a cancerous mole. The two roles – one professional and the other not - are not compatible.

I suppose we have always had this tension between the various roles of a pharmacist since the days of "alchemists" and "apothecaries" in ages past. It seems odd, however, that the arrangement still stands despite the advances that have been made in medical science as well as the dispelling of myths about how to treat illnesses and diseases.

If the tension between the professional and "non-professional" roles of the pharmacist was all I found unusual about pharmacy I think I could live with it. There are, however, other characteristics that seem incompatible with the professional image that pharmacists wish to present. These strengthen the impression that pharmacists do not know whether to stand tall as true health professionals or not.

The first example is the number of products of doubtful medical value that I find in some pharmacies. Homeopathic products come to mind. As far as I know these are equivalent to water; the difference being that they have a label to say that they contain a minuscule amount of some poison. Everybody agrees that there is no scientific basis for their use in a health service founded on science and that their perceived benefits can usually be attributed to a placebo effect.

Most professional bodies, including the Royal Pharmaceutical Society, think it is unethical to prescribe placebos. Despite this, there are lots of pharmacies that sell products such as these. When I have asked pharmacists why they stock them on their shelves, I have often been given the explanation that it is in the interest of promoting patient choice. This presents a problem for me. Patients want to have a choice on many things. Some would like to buy their alcohol, cigarettes and hard drugs from pharmacies. Surely a line has to be drawn somewhere.

In any case, there are "health stores" such as Holland and Barrett® that would arguably be more natural locations for such products. The inclusion of such products among proven therapies in pharmacies gives them a legitimacy that they perhaps have not earned.

This does not just apply to homeopathic products. Some of the common preparations we buy for coughs and colds are of doubtful benefit. When I had a cough some months ago my doctor advised against buying many of the popular brands, recommending instead one particular cheap generic formulation. This reduced my confidence in the products available for self-selection from pharmacies. Is it that pharmacists will sell anything "medical" if it drives their income? If so, are they any different from any other commercial enterprise whose sole driver is profit and whose minimum standard of ethical behaviour is what the law determines to be legal? I for one would prefer to be told by my pharmacist if an over the counter product was of doubtful value.

The second example is based on products that have absolutely no medicinal value and in fact promote a message contrary to what pharmacy is meant to represent. I have already mentioned "home brew" that some pharmacies (used to) sell. Pharmacists have a responsibility to advise patients how to drink responsibly. Most of them do so very well; using both opportunistic and targeted approaches to try to minimise inappropriate or excessive intake of alcohol. It seems odd for the pharmacies to then encourage the consumption of alcohol by selling kits to help patients brew beer at home. Admittedly there are few pharmacies that still do; but according to the media there is one large pharmacy chain in the United States that has taken a decision to sell some alcoholic beverages in some of its stores (Walgreens). Since this company is closely linked with one of the bigger chains in the UK (Boots), we can only hope that similar changes are not envisaged for this country.

Some people might think that alcohol is a bit far-fetched. Perhaps an example closer to home might illustrate the point. At the time of writing this book (early 2014); electronic cigarettes are still unlicensed products and they cannot be sold as nicotine replacement products. Legally they are just an alternative to regular cigarettes; in the sense that a person can choose to go for "full-strength" regular

cigarettes or opt for e-cigarettes that provide the same "hit" of nicotine without the tar and thousands of other nasty chemicals normally found in cigarettes. Electronic cigarettes have not undergone the rigorous testing that medicines – or standard nicotine replacement products – have undergone. Despite this, a lot of pharmacies now sell them. The pharmacists are not allowed to recommend them to people who wish to quit or reduce smoking; yet they sell them in the interest of "patient choice". It is hard to argue that such pharmacies would not sell regular cigarettes if this were deemed acceptable by the government.

This again beggars the question, "Are pharmacists health professionals that subscribe to clear codes of moral and ethical behaviour; or are they opportunistic retailers that sell whatever is profitable and legal in terms of the loosest interpretation of the laws that apply to them?"

The last evidence of an identity crisis is something that fascinated me at my last visit to the GP surgery a few weeks ago. Instead of seeing one of the regular GPs or prescribing nurses, I had a consultation with a part-time pharmacist. She did not just check my symptoms and issues with my regular repeat: she changed my medication completely. I was naturally surprised and asked if she was a "real" pharmacist. She responded that she was. She had just undertaken additional prescribing training. She tried to explain that she was not a doctor but as she was doing exactly the same things that my doctor does I was still confused when I left the surgery. I understand the role of pharmacists in manufacturing, dispensing and selling drugs, providing medical information, education or even in hospitals. However, moving into prescribing just muddies the water. How do I tell the difference between a pharmacist, a nurse and a doctor in that setting?

What exactly is a pharmacist?

Interrogations

After a relaxing evening in which I felt positive enough about pharmacy to suggest that pharmacists should be lead characters in dramas, I woke up to head into one of the bigger chains found on every high street up and down the country. With kids being on half-term break it was necessary to find an excuse to go out, even if it was to buy a packet of painkillers.

And so I walked into the shop, screaming kids in tow, and headed straight for the medicines counter.

"Can I help you?" asked the assistant in her most helpful voice.

"Yes please," I replied. *"May I have a packet of ABC painkillers?"*

As if a switch had flicked in her brain she automatically went into what I have now termed "Spanish Inquisition" mode:

"Who is this medicine for?"

"What are your symptoms?"

"How long have you used it for?"

"Are you on any other medicines?"

"What other medical conditions do you suffer from?"

I could repeat the script off by heart and I don't work behind the counter selling medicines every day. Surely the powers that be should understand how easy it is to rehearse your responses to these questions if you are really determined to get what you want. In any case, it is highly unlikely that a person of my age and gender will not be on some medication for one reason or another. I just don't feel like sharing that information when making even the most rudimentary of purchases of something I have used without harm for many years.

I am not addicted to ABC painkillers by the way. I only use them for very short periods thank you! In a way I feel patronised by such questions when I can easily get the same quantity of the painkillers from the local supermarket aisle without being asked a single question.

I understand the need for pharmacists and their teams to work to prevent inappropriate use of medicines; but there must be a better way of doing so. You need to balance concern about abuse and risk of harm from drugs against trusting that most intelligent, mature adults will be experienced in the safe use of common treatments. Somewhere between the "Spanish Inquisition" and unrestricted access is an acceptable solution.

Drug Addiction Services and Patient Confidentiality

Drug abuse is a scourge that has afflicted our society for a long time. Even Sir Arthur Conan Doyle's books about Sherlock Holmes, written in the 19th century, illustrate the abuse of opium and tobacco products. One of the great advances of medical science, in my view, has been the official acknowledgement of the risks associated with the use of tobacco, alcohol and other drugs.

Rarely is this more vividly exemplified than in the individuals that go to my local pharmacy for treatment for drug and alcohol addiction. You can usually tell a "drug addict" by the indicators of long-term use of drugs; namely a somewhat emaciated body frame, poor dental hygiene and an overall haggard look. This is by no means universal. There are some people who get treatment for drug addiction but otherwise look "normal". I use the term "drug addict" cautiously to refer to the stereotypical individual described above and undergoing treatment for addiction to illicit drugs. I shall consider over-the-counter drug addicts elsewhere.

I have conflicting views about the treatments and approaches taken towards drug addicts. On one hand I appreciate that these are just people that have made poor choices due to any combination of personal and domestic factors. The level of accountability for these choices undoubtedly varies depending on personal factors. Someone from an abusive home or relationship in a council estate, in which drug misuse is already a major problem, probably faces a more uphill struggle than another person from a "stereotypical" middle class suburban home. I admire doctors and pharmacists for the hope they offer individuals caught in the addiction trap through non-judgmental treatment of drug addiction.

My admiration is however tempered by concerns, fear, ignorance and possible prejudice. In the first instance I notice that in many pharmacies individuals with drug addiction problems are treated somewhat less equally than everyone else. I know that pharmacists will protest that they treat all patients equally but this does not seem to be true when some patients are expected to take their drugs in front of all other patients. When I walk into a pharmacy with my green prescription nobody knows whether it is for Viagra®, HRT tablets or treatment for Chlamydia. The pharmacist (normally) handles it very discreetly and gives me the products in a sealed bag thus respecting my need for confidentiality. If she needs to provide additional advice, she takes me to a side room and closes the door behind us so that nobody else can hear the discussion.

It seems that all these simple rules are thrown out of the window when it comes to drug addicts. First of all they are given a blue prescription that just screams, "I AM A DRUG ADDICT!" Secondly, on every occasion that the patient collects the medication, the pharmacist usually holds up the prescription and calls out the name of the patient to confirm the address and/or date of birth, thus announcing to the world that the person is collecting a drug for an addict or is an addict. Lastly if the patient is meant to be supervised they are often expected to take their "dose" in a section of the pharmacy that is visible to other "regular" patients. I have more than once seen parents in awkward situations in which their young children have asked why "that men is taking his medicines there".

Is this the way to treat someone who has realised his mistake and wants to come off drugs? It somehow feels as if we continue punishing people for crimes even after they have stopped using illicit drugs and their bodies have suffered for doing so. Some pharmacies provide a "privacy screen" to shield addicts as they drink their doses; whereas others have a dedicated room for the purpose. While I agree that these can be misconstrued as being solely "methadone" rooms (when they can be used for so much more), surely having some form of screen or room is better than having none at all.

I mentioned prejudice and fear as other barriers. From a patient perspective I have to be honest that I used to avoid some pharmacies due to the numbers of "drug addicts" they served. I had a fear of being robbed or ill-treated in some way. Some of my friends and acquaintances still do. This is unfortunate because most recovering drug addicts are decent individuals that are not going to attempt to rob you at first sight. What is inexcusable though is the attitude of some pharmacists and pharmacies towards addicts. I do not think I'm the only one who has noticed that there are certain pharmacies that do not welcome recovering drug addicts. Recovering drug addicts are disproportionately underrepresented in some supermarket, edge-of-town or high street pharmacies.

My last observation about drug addiction services relates to needle and syringe services run from pharmacies. I find puzzling the fact that active illicit drug users can go into a pharmacy and get needles, syringes, pans, filters and citric acid – the works – on demand. It is evident that such requests are to facilitate the injection of illicit street heroin, yet it is perfectly legal to supply "works" for this purpose.

On one hand pharmacies are actively promoting abstinence from drug abuse coupled with services to facilitate recovery; on the other they facilitate illicit drug use. This seems, at best, very odd. Perhaps the need for easy access to "clean works" – easily met through community pharmacies – trumps any such concerns.

Pharmacy Surveys

In an earlier chapter I wrote about the questions that are asked at most pharmacies whenever you are buying any medicines.

I had just undergone the interrogation discussed before when, as I was about to walk away from the counter, the assistant said in her most cheery voice,

"Would you like to do one of our surveys, please? You just go to this website and you could win this and that. This is the code you need to enter."

She pointed at a long number on the piece of paper.

Perhaps my experience is unique; but I gather too much rubbish in the form of receipts when I go shopping. The first thing I want to do when I get home is to safely dispose of these receipts to make room for more important things. If I am on a shopping trip and I visit three or four stores, one of which is a chemist, I am unlikely to get home and search through my receipts just to find the one from the chemist so I can complete a survey. All the major retailers have these survey invitations printed on their receipts. If I do one then I have to do all of them.

A pharmacy would need to really stand out for me to make the time for the survey. I suspect I am not the only person with this "problem". The rate of return on patient survey invitations handed out to customers to fill in at home must be depressingly low. I sympathise with the poor souls that have to ask customers to fill in the surveys day in and day out. I also dread to think of the number of trees that are destroyed to make the paper wasted on these receipts. A more efficient and environmentally-friendly way of getting the responses is needed.

Perhaps the answer can be found in both low- and high-tech solutions. My surgery employs a low-tech but highly effective option. Once a year the practice undertakes a survey asking for feedback from patients about how it has done over the previous year. It prints several hundred paper copies of the questionnaire and leaves them in the waiting area for patients to fill in whilst waiting for their appointments. It also asks local pharmacies to take some copies and hand them out to customers to fill in whilst waiting for their prescriptions to be dispensed. The completed questionnaires are then collected and analysed at the surgery. This seems like a simple but effective solution. Why do pharmacies not ask patients to fill out questionnaires while waiting for their prescriptions? This would provide a more accurate snapshot of patient views at the time of service provision.

The high-tech solution might be in the form of a touch-screen device in the pharmacy (secured to an immovable base station) that provides access to an electronic version of the survey. Again this would offer the chance to get immediate feedback and reduce the resources and time needed. Both alternatives also offer a distinct advantage in comparison with the current method: I would probably only be asked once in a long while to complete the survey; something that I think I could live with."

Besides the mechanisms of completing the surveys as requested, I also have concerns about the reasons and variations in the surveys available from different pharmacies. Some pharmacy teams are honest enough to state that they have to get a certain number of responses as part of their contract, that they genuinely use the feedback as a basis for improving their services and that the "bosses" demand that they get a specified number of responses.

What I still find puzzling are the variations in the questions asked when you complete surveys from different companies. One might ask if you have a loyalty card, have heard about the electronic prescription service, how many members are in your family or several other questions that are not asked by another. This not only elongates and reduces the likelihood of completing the survey; it reduces the enthusiasm for completing surveys in future.

It also raises the question, "What exactly are pharmacies meant to ask in the survey?"

If there is a legal requirement to ask certain questions, these should be identical across all the pharmacies, with an option at the end to answer additional optional questions tailored for each pharmacy or chain. That way we can give pharmacies the basic answers they need to meet their legal obligations; and then, for the chance to win any of the prizes they advertise, voluntarily answer any other additional questions if interested.

Pharmacy Services and Patient Signatures

On the 16th of October, 2013 I published a post on my blog questioning the need to sign for so many things whenever I speak to the pharmacist. Since publishing the post I have learnt that pharmacists really do need to have my signature not only to prove that they have obtained my permission to undertake a "Medicines Use Review,"

"Appliance Use Review" or "New Medicine Service"; but also to allow the NHS authorities to access my records to verify that the pharmacies are not committing fraud by claiming for services they have not undertaken!

It's a tough life for pharmacists: Not only do they have to deal with distrustful patients like me; even their paymasters do not trust them as professionals. This is a bit disconcerting. However, when you delve a bit deeper into the world of pharmacy and read the conversations among pharmacists, you find that money has been getting taken away from the traditional dispensing services that pharmacies provide and the only way to get it back is to undertake these services. There is a small temptation to fiddle the figures among dishonest pharmacists. I guess that's a discussion for another day.

Anyway, here's the text for my blog post from the 16th of October, 2013:

"I like to think I have a good professional relationship with my local chemist – or pharmacist as she likes to point out. I trust her to give me the correct medication for my many conditions and she, well, she somehow makes money from the process. I don't yet fully understand how she does this but I'm in the process of finding out.

My pharmacist has worked at the pharmacy for over ten. I remember when she first arrived and took over from "Mr Burns" – bubbling with energy and keen to use her clinical knowledge. It seems that age, or life experience, has dampened her enthusiasm somewhat.

I also recall the first time that she took me into the small room for a "chat about my regular medicines". This must be going back all of seven or eight years. She took in all of her big pharmacy reference books and asked me to bring all my medication from my house. I knew about the appointment a fortnight in advance and we spent nearly an hour discussing not just my medicines but my understanding of my underlying conditions and when, why or how I took each of my medicines. She must have gone through every side effect checking to see that I was not experiencing any of them. She had reams of paper on which she recorded everything about me. To be frank I felt a bit frightened afterwards and somewhat overloaded with information. She also gave me lots of paperwork that I was meant to read. I honestly do not recall reading any of it but I can't remember exactly where it disappeared to. I suspect, like most papers I do not need, it found its way to the recycling bin.

Every year since then she has made sure that we have our "annual chat". Not surprisingly these chats have got shorter and shorter because the doctor only ever changes one or two of my drugs, if at all, in-between the chats. I am lucky to get five minutes where I got nearly an hour seven years ago. I often wonder what the point of the annual chats is. Surely I'm not so forgetful that I need to be reminded every year what my regular medication is for. On the other hand, I feel that perhaps I am not cared for as much as I was less than a decade ago. Is it that my pharmacist has lost the caring side that made her willing to spend so much time with me in the past; or is she under pressure to limit the time that she spends with each of her patients?

I have also noticed over the past couple of years that whenever we have these "chats" she asks me to sign a piece of paper confirming that we have indeed held the conversation. This never used to be the case. Is it that she has been found to be untrustworthy and thus has to prove to her bosses/the NHS/whoever that she is not making things up? Is it a requirement for pharmacists to have written permission for every conversation they have with patients? If the authorities do not trust her to be honest about this, how can they expect patients to trust her professionalism? It also seems like pharmacists get a bit of a raw deal compared with other health professionals. How is it that I don't have to sign a piece of paper whenever I visit my GP but have to do so at the pharmacy?

Having to sign these pieces of paper really does get in the way of building trust. Sometimes it feels like the signature was the only thing that the pharmacist wanted in the first place."

Public Relations and Community Pharmacy

My pharmacist likes to tell me that patients visit pharmacies much more than they visit the GP or nurse, yet many of us see pharmacists as little more than specialist shopkeepers. My personal acquaintance with the profession has been a bit of a learning curve that has only been made possible by the relationship I have with my pharmacist and some deliberate attempts I made to understand the profession.

A few years ago, to my embarrassment, I came to the realisation that I knew very little about pharmacy. I used to have a rather transactional relationship with the local pharmacist. I got a piece of paper from the doctor or dentist with an order for some medicine and directions on how to use it; took this to the pharmacy for processing and left with a bag containing the right stuff. Doctors prescribed and pharmacists dispensed medicines. I also frequented the pharmacy for tissues, toiletries and other things.

This view was in a way shaped by the perception that if I were really ill I would make an appointment to see the doctor; but if I wanted to buy something I could go to the pharmacy, the supermarket or even the local garage; depending on whichever was most convenient at the time. The first chapter in this book talks about the pharmacy identity crisis, summarising my impressions until recently on what pharmacy stood for.

I am not alone among patients in being somewhat bemused by this group of professionals that are found on every high street. This is reflected in the terminology used to refer to them. Here in the UK a lot of people refer to pharmacists as "chemists"; whereas in parts of the US pharmacies are referred to as "drugstores", which is not too dissimilar to our old word, "druggist". All these terms reflect the understanding of the pharmacist's role as that of compounding and selling medicines, usually in accordance with a doctor's directions.

Several months ago I decided to "follow" a few pharmacists and pharmacy technicians on Twitter® and the blogosphere. I started with some popular pharmacy celebrities such as Mr Dispenser, author of two books under the common title, "Pills, Thrills and Methadone Spills;" then followed other key "celebrities" such as @MrDodgyChemist and an American pharmacist by the name @CrazyRxMan. These gave me a flavour of the world of pharmacy both in the UK and North America. This was followed by more people from both the UK and the US, with my preference being UK-based professionals. I deliberately chose to do a lot more listening than talking.

In the process I gained a fair understanding of the language of pharmacy and what the job of a pharmacist entails. In fact, I picked up a few terms and could speak so intelligently about pharmacy that some friends started asking if I had ever worked in a pharmacy myself. What I have learnt has shown me the following about pharmacists.

Firstly, pharmacists are very good at talking to each other about job-related issues and even about patients. Some of them even poke fun at us patients in much the same way I imagine those who work in restaurants must do whenever they get an awkward customer. They use social media to share anecdotes about work and to highlight something wrong that they have come across; be it a wrongly-written prescription or a misunderstanding about the trials and tribulations of their job. Reading their interactions with each other almost felt like spying, from a clandestine post, on a conclave of believers.

I wish pharmacists made more of an effort to interact with the rest of us "non-pharmacy" people. I get the fact that most of the Twitter accounts I followed were of a personal nature and the owners did not see themselves as having a "public relations" role for pharmacy; but it struck me as odd that even when I raised issues of interest on my blog none of them would respond publicly; although admittedly I got one or two retweets and some of my tweets were "favourited".

I also acknowledge that some pharmacists have written books meant for patients to understand the world of pharmacy. However, other than Jemima McCandless, the author of the book "Confessions of a Chemist", the others I have read have been published under pseudonyms.

The second observation is that pharmacists appear to live in an atmosphere of fear: fear of bosses, patients, the NHS police, lawyers, employers, colleagues or even employees. This is reflected in the nature of the posts and the names adopted by the professionals on their blogs and on Twitter®. The most popular and satirical (some would say honest) blogs and profiles are those in which the owners have assumed a screen persona for the purpose of purveying their views (Mr Dispenser, Mr Dodgy Dispenser, Crazy RxMan etc). This suggests that there are consequences to honesty. Pharmacists rely on the relative anonymity of social media to provide an outlet for the frustrations of their job. (Mr Dispenser is admittedly an exception in this regard as he is said to have made an appearance in person at the Pharmacy Show in 2013 for an official book-signing ceremony. His Twitter® profile indicates that he is currently on a tour of pharmacy schools across the UK hence he is not really "anonymous" in the same sense as the other pharmacists. I must add that he is not among the most controversial of the Twitter profiles from what I can see.)

I know what you're thinking: How come I also use a pseudonym?. Well, check out my blog for the answer to that question.

Going back to pharmacists, the third observation is that pharmacists desperately need some form of coordinated public relations effort at communicating with the public with one voice and reminding us how valuable they are to sustaining our quality of life. I have come across many different pharmacy organisations and "voices", but I am still uncertain which one can claim to be representative of pharmacy when it speaks. Compare this with doctors. When the British Medical Association speaks, you know that it is speaking on behalf of doctors and what it says is listened to by the government and the public alike.

Pharmacists, on the other hand, are represented by the National Pharmacy Association, Pharmaceutical Services Negotiating Committee, Independent Pharmacists' Federation, Company Chemists Association, Association of Independent Multiple Pharmacies and the Royal Pharmaceutical Society; and that's only the ones I know about. In the past couple of years it appears that pharmacists have realised the problems associated with having so many different viewpoints and some of them have come up with something called "Pharmacy Voice". This however only represents three of the bodies listed above; and it seems to be very good at providing responses to documents, government initiatives, publications and proposals. It has not made a concerted effort at engaging with patients but instead seems to be more interested in talking to the government, or more specifically those referred to as the "NHS paymasters" in the pharmacy world.

As it stands, it appears that "Pharmacy Voice" is just a coordinated opinion mouthpiece for the three organisations; but does not have any clout in negotiating for the member organisations or speaking to the public on behalf of the profession. In any case, the name "Pharmacy Voice" comes across as trying a bit too hard and fails to adequately depict what the organisation represents. We know that word "pharmacy" refers to much more than the experience of retails pharmacists. For "Pharmacy Voice" to be truly meaningful it would have to represent the views of pharmacists across all sectors of practice and all sizes of organisation.

Medicine Wastage

I have been at a pharmacy on more than one occasion when a patient or representative has brought in a large carrier or bin bag full of medicines that have not been used. I am always shocked at this. One day I felt that I could not help asking the pharmacist (once the patient had left and there was nobody else nearby) a few questions about patient-returned medicines. I felt that there had to be a way to reduce the wastage.

On the one hand I understand the value of the service that pharmacies provide in taking back any unused medicines. If people were unable to return their unused drugs I suppose the majority would flush them down the toilet or dispose of them with their domestic waste. I do not think that our domestic water treatment works are engineered to deal with the large range of drugs that people take, from drugs for cancer to hormones in the common pill. Since waste water is partially recycled for drinking in some parts of the world, I can imagine that we would see an increase in harmful effects if drugs and medicines were not properly disposed of on a large scale. Pharmacists perform a useful function in this sense.

41

This does not mean that I understand where exactly drugs go once they have been left with the pharmacist. I would like to imagine that the pharmacist does not pour them down the drain on our behalf!

On a more serious note, when I asked the pharmacist if the medicines were recycled for use by other patients I was told that this has not been allowed for many years. My mother tells me of a time when you could recycle even your empty tablet containers so as to minimise wastage; but my pharmacist indicates that it is now considered unethical to collect patient-returned medicines for donation to developing countries where there might be drug shortages; something that used to be done until relatively recently.

I quickly asked for some clarification and bombarded the pharmacist with further questions.

The first problem I had was with the amount of drugs that people do not use and consequently have to return to a pharmacy. I asked for an approximate indication of the value of unused medication returned by patients in an average month. The pharmacist could not give me a figure as he indicated that they do not have the resources to monitor the value of patient-returned drugs. What he did show me though was a large yellow bin that he said weighed an average of about twenty kilograms (3 stone 2 pounds). He said that over a three month period his pharmacy filled anywhere between eight and fifteen of these huge bins. These were then collected by specialist waste companies for incineration at high temperatures.

Working on an average of six bins per pharmacy every quarter, I estimated that there would be about 69,000 such bins or nearly one thousand four hundred tonnes of wasted medicines per quarter in England alone. I suppose truly accurate figures can only be obtained from these specialist waste companies. I also realise that any figures that are available are based solely on medicines returned to pharmacies. Nobody knows how many medicines still end up in the bin or down the drain at the homes of patients.

Whilst the mass of wasted drugs is shocking by any standard, I decided to do an online search to find out if anyone had ever attempted to estimate the cost of such wasted medicines. There is a Guardian article from the 3rd of July 2012 that estimates that about £150 million worth of drugs are wasted this way every year. This is upsetting as it suggests that as a nation we are effectively letting that much money go up in smoke since such drugs have to be destroyed once they return to the pharmacy.

This leads me to a second problem. When I probed further why patient-returned drugs could not be recycled even though they appeared to be in good condition and the packaging was fully intact, the pharmacist explained that pharmacists have a professional responsibility to ensure that any medication they supply for use by a patient has been stored under appropriate conditions of temperature, humidity and light, in addition to not being adulterated or tempered with in any way since the point of manufacture. Providing this assurance is straightforward if the drug has been in the pharmaceutical supply chain but once it leaves the pharmacy for a patient's home this becomes impossible.

The pharmacist gave me an example based on the fact that some people store their medicines in the bathroom or in a kitchen with fluctuating temperatures; all of which could reduce the efficacy of the drugs by reducing their potency. I could not argue against this; hence I asked when the profession and government had fist realised that it was a significant problem. Had there been complaints from developing countries about donated drugs not being effective? Had actual tests been carried out on representative samples of patient-returned drugs to prove that the concerns were founded? Could the arguments not actually have originated from manufacturing companies that wanted to protect their markets in developing countries by preventing free supplies of needed medication from reaching the poor; from developed countries?

The pharmacist understandably indicated that he was not able to answer these questions as he did not have the necessary background information. He was however bound by legal constraints to comply with the guidelines on how to deal with such drugs; and I was not about to encourage him to break the law.

The third concern I had with such drugs centred on the patient end of the problem. It struck me that we patients have a responsibility not to waste both drugs and money the way we currently do (well, those that do). Many of us take the NHS for granted either because we do not pay directly for the privilege of using it or because we pay a reduced fee in terms of the prescription charge. I think if we paid directly for the cost of treatment – as some people do in other countries – we would be less likely to waste medicines, dressings and whatever else we get on the NHS.

This of course raises a related question: Could it be that the reason there is so much wastage is that people simply do not understand or think about the cost of their treatment? This is possible. The problem is how to address this in such a way that it changes people's behaviour positively. Human psychology being what it is, I do not think that simply telling people that they are on expensive medication will solve the problem. Innovative ways of assuring patients that they are on effective medication that should be taken/used as directed have to be found.

My suggestion is that any patient education program on avoiding drug wastage should focus on people's sense of decency and the common good; more of a nudge towards doing what is right than a push. Achieving this will call for some innovative approaches; but it certainly can be done. It has to be done.

Problems with appreciating the cost of drugs

I have been in the embarrassing situation in which I thought my pharmacy had given me wrong medication and I went back to the pharmacy in a huff to get this corrected. I was used to one particular brand and so when I got a different drug I was convinced that an error had been made. It took quite a lot of explaining for the pharmacist to explain that I was getting the same active component as I had been getting for several years the only difference was that I was getting what is referred to as its generic equivalent, now that the brand had come off-patent.

I reluctantly accepted the explanation and decided to give the 'new' version a try. Thankfully I was pleasantly surprised to find that it worked. Perhaps there are people out there in similar shoes.

Let me explain. If I have a medical condition and am told that there are two possible comparable treatments for my condition, one of which is much more expensive than the other, I will in most cases opt for the more expensive treatment, especially if somebody else is paying (i.e. the

47

NHS). The common assumption is that "if it's cheap, then it's not as good." I guess this is why doctors struggle to explain to patients that the perceived marginal benefits of a "new" treatment do not justify the massive difference in cost, whenever a new wonder drug or treatment comes to market. One doctor friend has cynically highlighted how these differences tend to become less significant as the patent expiry dates of such new drugs approach.

The same logic applies to the brand versus generic drug debate. As in my case, patients assume that branded drugs are always better than generic equivalents, as reflected in the price. Health professionals will of course know the absurdity of this assumption, since long-standing treatments become cheaper once their patents expire and they can be mass-produced by a larger number of manufacturers using more economical methods. I imagine that pharmacists have a hard time explaining this to patients though.

The second problem associated with an appreciation of the true cost of drugs is that it increases the temptation among some people to make a quick buck. Only a few weeks ago people tried to flog off their smartphones for thousands of pounds on eBay when they found out that the manufacturer of one popular game had withdrawn the game from the market. I can easily see some people with non-life-threatening conditions and on expensive drugs being similarly tempted to sell drugs both off and online. Examples might be people on growth hormone injections (popular with body builders) or certain strong painkillers.

A third concern might arise from the opposite problem: drugs being comparatively cheap. My pharmacist has often reminded me that the prescription charge I pay is an NHS levy, not a payment for the cost of drugs. Hence, although I pay the standard prescription charge for some antibiotics, their true cost can be less than a pound. If this were to become widely known among prescription-paying patients, more would ask for such cheap drugs to be issued on private prescription; and for expensive drugs to be issued on NHS prescriptions, thus resulting in the NHS losing out.

Perhaps there's a case to be made for too much information not being given to the public when it comes to certain issues.

My Suggestions for Community Pharmacy

(Note: This chapter is entirely an opinion piece on how I think community pharmacy could be improved for pharmacists and patients alike. I wish to thank all the pharmacists that contributed towards the final product by giving their views and corrections on my understanding of the community pharmacy contract. A lot of them did not agree with my views but they thought it a good idea to include them in the book to stimulate further debate. I asked for their feedback on condition of anonymity and will respect my commitments to them. My gratitude knows no bounds. I do of course retain responsibility for any errors that remain.)

We are all aware that pharmacists are very good at their role in the supply chain. They efficiently source drugs and supply them against prescriptions. At the same time they sell many other products without prescription. However, it is accepted both within and outside the profession that most of the supply component is an under-utilisation of the pharmacists' skills. It is something that can be mechanised (hence dispensers and dispensing robots); subject to the involvement of the pharmacist in checking the clinical suitability of the prescriptions. Yet it seems that most pharmacists in the country are tied to dispensing stations in pharmacies.

Let's look at this in depth. I credit one of my pharmacist friends for the following analysis. The typical pharmacy is essentially no different to a factory. We have inputs (prescriptions and the pre-packed boxes of tablets or liquids), machinery and units of production (computers, software, labels, pens etc.), human resources (dispensers) and outputs (packaged medicines with labels on them). Most of the prescriptions that the typical pharmacy handles are for "repeat" medicines; hence processing them is relatively straightforward. In these situations one is tempted to see a typical pharmacy as not very different from a fast-food outlet such as McDonalds ® or KFC®. The processes involved are repetitive and easily replicable. Whenever we have such processes the result is that the value we place on them declines.

In economics terms, the marginal value of each dispensing operation is so low that pharmacies have to chase large volumes of prescriptions in order to generate sufficient turnover to operate profitably. This works well if a process is entirely mechanised, but human beings don't scale up as well as machines do. Humans have finite capabilities and the result of increasing prescription volumes will only be an increase in the stress levels experienced by individual pharmacists. Errors might increase and pharmacists would consequently be sued.

In a world in which there are limited resources for funding pharmacy within the NHS, retail pharmacy will either have to mechanise or find a way to pay less for most of the processes associated with dispensing. Sadly this means that pharmacists face a downward pressure on their earnings as prescription volumes increase. Recent discussions in the pharmacy world indicate that the numbers of pharmacy graduates being churned out from the universities are increasing, a factor that can only result in further downward pressures on pharmacist salaries in line with the principles of demand and supply.

Although the reduction in payments for pharmacy services seems to be a positive thing for the NHS and patients, my worry as a patient is that a low-paid profession will eventually attract low-calibre candidates and result in

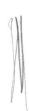

poor pharmacists. Alternatively it might mean that the profession fails to innovate in ways that would otherwise have benefitted us all in future.

In order for pharmacists to progress, therefore, it is important that they realise that their failure to dissociate themselves from the dispensing process is only going to drive their earnings downwards. For most retail pharmacists this spells doom since they have no "get-out" option. They are employees beholden to large and small chains that hold the "contracts" for the operation of pharmacies. The individual pharmacists themselves do not have contracts with the NHS, but their employers do. As a result, the pharmacists can easily be replaced without major impacts on the operations. Once such pharmacists are unemployed, it is difficult for them to get their own contracts for pharmacies; or to otherwise find ways of profitably making use of their skills.

Associated with this is the realisation that the aims of the contractor-employer are not necessarily aligned with those of the typical employee-pharmacist. It is to be expected that in most cases the former will prevail over the latter. There are also implications for the nature of the pharmacy contract itself. Does the contract reflect patient needs, pharmacist abilities and skills, or simply what the NHS has said it is willing to pay for and which also is seen as commercially viable by contractors?

Compare this with nurses and doctors. Nurses are largely employed by hospitals. Their situation is very similar to pharmacists, with one key difference: they are mostly in the public sector whereas pharmacists are in the private sector. The public sector has a primary purpose to provide services for the good of the public whereas the private sector seeks firstly to make a profit for the owners/shareholders. Nurses have, as a result, been able to expand their roles much more rapidly than have pharmacists. It could be said that nurses arguably utilise more of their skills than do pharmacists. It appears therefore that the "employee" status of pharmacists results in their progression in utilising their skills being entirely dependent on the wishes of the employers, not on patients or directly on the pharmacists themselves.

Again, if we compare pharmacists with GPs, we find interesting differences. Both are in the private sector but, without a doubt, the individual GP is much more successful than the pharmacist. We have already said that in retail

54

pharmacy the employer generally holds the contract, and the pharmacist is there to facilitate the provision of the services under the contract. The biggest pharmacy chain in the UK, Boots®, commands more than twenty per cent of the market share. GPs, on the other hand, still operate under what has been described as a cottage industry. This is made up of individual GPs and small groups of GPs that hold contracts with the NHS and are directly represented by the relevant professional body.

In other words, the body that represents the contractors represents the professionals, and the wishes of the contractor and those of the professionals are virtually the same. GPs are able to commission services directly and their scope for professional practice is to a large extent dependent on how far they are willing to utilise the full scope of their professional training. The GMS contract is structured to reflect the abilities of the GPs. This is important as it means that GPs can influence their contract in better ways than pharmacists. This allows a scope for innovation among GPs that pharmacists cannot hope to replicate.

Perhaps this is reflected in the disparity of earnings between GPs and pharmacists. Some pharmacists argue that whereas the "salary" of an individual pharmacist a few decades ago was comparable to that of a typical GP, nowadays it is anywhere between half and a third of the latter. I have discussed the role of the different contracts above. As indicated before, not everybody agrees with this view. Some people argue that the change is attributable to the move from individual contractors to multiples controlling the pharmacy market.

One piece of evidence in favour of this view, they argue, is that employee GPs earn roughly half of what contractor GPs earn. In fact, the salary of an employee GP is not too different from that of an experienced employee pharmacist.

For pharmacists to improve their standing, they should work towards a situation in which they hold the contracts for the services that they provide. Some pharmacists have been clamouring for a return to the days when they held the contracts for the dispensing operations. However, as a patient I do not see this as providing justification for pharmacists being well-paid. As indicated above, the actual dispensing process, as a supply operation, does not merit high earnings.

I think pharmacists ought to be seen to be adding value to the dispensing process. This might be through community pharmacists, for instance, performing a more intensive clinical assessment role on prescriptions. I think pharmacists would agree with me that they are hampered in achieving this outside the GP surgery as they do not have access to the full medical records for the patients that they come across. One way around this would be for pharmacists to offer prescription assessment services to GP surgeries. This would involve checking the suitability of all prescriptions generated against the other medicines on record, the patient's age and overall suitability in terms of the dose and the duration of the course. I expect that GP prescribing systems offer something along these lines but what I see on Twitter® indicates that a lot of wrong prescriptions still slip through the net.

Such pharmacist services as suggested above can be done under current arrangements without any changes to infrastructure or technological changes. I suspect that any challenges relate to finding an additional room for a pharmacist within the surgery. I can also imagine that the process would lengthen prescription-processing times. This would not go down well with patients and dispensing pharmacies.

There is probably a better option: ensuring that pharmacists have full access to a patient's medication history directly from within the pharmacy. Checking freshly-generated prescriptions against GP records in surgeries might not be adequate in preventing medication problems since patients often take a lot of other medicines that they obtain directly from pharmacies without notifying their GPs. I am not sure how significant such purchases are since patients do not just buy medicines from pharmacies. As indicated in an earlier chapter I get mine from the supermarket or local garage as well.

I sometimes wonder if it is really necessary for the pharmacist to be on the pharmacy premises. Is it not possible, for instance, to have a computerized system of checking whether drugs on a prescription are suitable for a patient based on their other medication? My friends in pharmacy tell me that their patient medication systems already do that. However, the systems do not give a straightforward "yes" or "no" indication about whether to issue a drug or not. Someone has to make a clinical decision based on the available information about a drug's profile, the patient's conditions, personal characteristics and medication history. That decision falls on the pharmacist within the community pharmacy setting.

This realization is part of what gives me confidence in community pharmacy; knowing that there is a competent professional to review my treatment right at the point of provision. It is also why I think it a good idea for pharmacists to have access to my medication history. On a wider scale I can imagine that pharmacies must face challenges in getting full and accurate information from some patients at times. Some customers could either choose not to tell the full truth about their medical history or simply not remember their specific medication names when asked by the pharmacy teams. The decision not to disclose full details need not arise from abuse of drugs: I would not wish to tell the assistant at the till that I was on Viagra® or HRT in front of other customers whilst making a quick purchase.

The problem that pharmacists in community pharmacists have, in my view, is that they do not get enough time for these other professional assessments that only they can do; that and the fact that the contracts for various services seem to be with the contractors and not necessarily the pharmacists. Part of the reason for the former is that pharmacists are too tied up in the dispensing process. Community pharmacy needs to find a way of freeing pharmacists from the dispensing process by having robust clinical checking systems.

I dare say that changes could be taken a step further. Once pharmacists have been freed in this way then they could possibly get individual contracts for professional services based on their interests, specialities and local demand. I am aware that pharmacists already provide medicines use reviews and the new medicine service. However, you only need to look up the discussions on pharmacy forums and social media to know that for many pharmacists this has become a "numbers game" under pressure from managers and employers. Quality is sacrificed under the pressure to check large volumes of prescriptions whilst doing a million other things that pharmacists are expected to attend to but which they arguably do not really need to do. I suspect that pharmacists with this level of autonomy would also be able to introduce new services that would benefit patients and the NHS alike.

I expect that current contractors and large multiples will balk at the idea of losing control of their pharmacists and, more importantly, the contracts. However, this need not necessarily result in doom and gloom for the likes of Boots® and Lloyds®. Existing pharmacies have built up extremely efficient operations around dispensing. Tinkering with these unnecessarily will result in the introduction of inefficiencies and drive up costs. On the other hand, the pharmacy forums make it clear that existing pharmacies often struggle to incorporate the range of additional services that are part of the pharmacy contract; and few pharmacies actually provide the full range of services available under their contract.

Allowing for pharmacists to be commissioned to provide services in their own capacity might "incentivize" pharmacists to provide more services. This would benefit patients, the pharmacists themselves and owners of pharmacy premises. It need not disrupt the experience for patients. The owners of premises from which dispensing services are provided would retain the right to "rent out" the premises to the pharmacists that hold the services contracts. Pharmacists would have to go where the patients were.

Some might choose GP surgeries. Most, I suspect, would choose the more familiar pharmacy setting.

It also seems a fairer system of rewarding professionals than a straight wage. There might scope for pharmacists and owners of premises reaching agreements on the relative distribution of the professional services payments.

It would also be possible, at least in theory, for pharmacists to set up their own premises from which to provide services. That would of course create the challenge of attracting patients to such premises and explaining how they differ from "conventional" pharmacies. Opportunity however, like necessity, can be a strong driver of inventiveness.

In summary, the benefits of reviewing the pharmacy contract and placing a greater emphasis on the pharmacists' professional skills would be as follows:

Firstly, there are benefits for pharmacists from a professional viewpoint. They would be able to utilise their skills in accordance with their qualifications. This would promote the development of new services and develop retail pharmacy in ways that have not been possible before. In the process, it would force pharmacists to continuously improve their competence in line with the demands of the services that they need to provide. Pharmacists would be freed from what they perceive as the "unprofessional" pressure that they feel they sometimes face from some managers and owners to play the numbers game. In addition, it would also make it easier for them to be directly accountable for the services they provide in a manner akin to that of doctors and other health professionals. Finally, it would also create opportunities for community pharmacists to expand their services to GP surgeries and thus work in association with other health professionals.

From the perspective of regulators and the NHS it would create clear lines of accountability for different aspects of pharmacy operations. Issues of pharmacy staffing levels and premises standards would be taken up with dispensing contractors; whilst services would directly be the responsibility of pharmacists. It might actually create further cost savings in payments for dispensing services. In cases of fraud it would be easy for the regulators to question dispensing contractors over prescription declarations; while queries over services would be addressed by questioning the pharmacist contractors that made the relevant declarations. There are also potential savings if pharmacists are freed up to have proper chats with patients about medicines, potentially leading to reductions in wastage through unused medicines. Finally, it would create a unique opportunity for some joined-up thinking by linking the GP and pharmacy contracts, since both professions are meant to be working for the benefit of patients.

For patients the benefits might involve faster services from pharmacies; but mainly they would involve benefitting from new or properly-conducted services. Problems with prescribed medicines, such as non-adherence, excessive quantities on prescription and side effects would be identified earlier and addressed. These in turn would lead to a reduction in wasted medication or unnecessary hospital admissions.

There are of course some challenges to the implementation of the plan. The first one is that not all pharmacists are attracted to the idea of becoming contractors. It is likely that a lot prefer being employee pharmacists with a guaranteed stable salary at the end of the month. This should still be possible within the suggested framework. Pharmacists could take a leaf from GPs in this regard. Although GPs generally work in partnerships; it is not unheard of to have an employee GP within the practice – one who has passed the training but is either not willing to be or not yet at the level of a partner. Lawyers, accountants, architects and other professionals also have similar arrangements. The employee pharmacists could either work for pharmacist services or dispensing contractors, depending on their preference. They would just have to be willing to accept lower wages in the process.

The second challenge is that in practice it is unlikely that there will ever be a time when there is no need for a pharmacist at some stage of the dispensing process. Within the dispensing environment there is often an unpredictable need for a pharmacist. By this I mean that there are times when a pharmacist might need to be called upon without prior warning. If a patient comes in with a query on a clinical issue related to a prescription that has just been dispensed; or another one makes a phone call about a prescription drug; then a pharmacist needs to be on hand to deal with the query. In addition, patients can walk into the pharmacy and present with symptoms that require a pharmacist's evaluation to determine whether it should be symptomatically treated in the pharmacy or referred to the doctor (or the hospital). One of the attractions of community pharmacy is the ready accessibility of the pharmacist; which facilitates counter-prescribing and the signposting of patients to appropriate health care services. If this aspect of community pharmacy is removed, the knock-on effect will be more inappropriate self-referrals by patients to GPs and hospital A&E departments.

The final challenge is on the viability (read "profitability") of pharmacy services. Under current arrangements pharmacy incomes are largely derived from dispensing operations. Income from services is limited by the nature of the pharmacy contract. Pharmacists can only undertake a maximum of four hundred medicines use reviews at £28 each. Payment for the new medicines service is structured in bands and has a maximum limit. The funding for pharmaceutical services and dispensing operations is also constrained within the NHS; and the government is unlikely to be willing to increase it just to satisfy pharmacists' demands for increased funding for services.

In response I would suggest that the savings from "freeing" pharmacists from dispensing operations could be channelled to services. This could be vehemently opposed by dispensing contractors, all of whom are already feeling the pain from regular government cuts in payments for drugs under what is known as Category M price reductions. I suspect the overall level of opposition would depend on the balance between the funds that were being "diverted" this way towards services and the savings that were being made through efficiencies made in dispensing, such as through dispensing robots. (I've just made enemies among dispensers.)

If the idea of diverting funding this way appears ludicrous, it does not change the validity of the fundamental question: Is it a proper use of the pharmacists' skills to tie them to dispensing operations and reward them principally for this, when they are capable of so much more – or so we are led to believe? It can also be argued that the idea behind the latest changes to the NHS structures, including the creation of clinical commissioning groups. Provide an opportunity for any qualified group of professionals to introduce new, cost-effective and beneficial services for patients. Pharmacists have as much a right in this as anybody else.

All in all I think it's an idea worth taking a look at. It will certainly benefit patients, pharmacists and, ultimately, the government and the NHS.

Section 2: The GP Surgery

"I swear by Apollo, the healer, Asclepius, Hygieia, and Panacea, and I take to witness all the gods, all the goddesses, to keep according to my ability and my judgment, the following Oath and agreement:

To consider dear to me, as my parents, him who taught me this art; to live in common with him and, if necessary, to share my goods with him; To look upon his children as my own brothers, to teach them this art; and that by my teaching, I will impart a knowledge of this art to my own sons, and to my teacher's sons, and to disciples bound by an indenture and oath according to the medical laws, and no others.

I will prescribe regimens for the good of my patients according to my ability and my judgment and never do harm to anyone.

I will give no deadly medicine to any one if asked, nor suggest any such counsel; and similarly I will not give a woman a pessary to cause an abortion.

But I will preserve the purity of my life and my arts.

I will not cut for stone, even for patients in whom the disease is manifest; I will leave this operation to be performed by practitioners, specialists in this art.

In every house where I come I will enter only for the good of my patients, keeping myself far from all intentional ill-doing and all seduction and especially from the pleasures of love with women or men, be they free or slaves.

All that may come to my knowledge in the exercise of my profession or in daily commerce with men, which ought not to be spread abroad, I will keep secret and will never reveal.

If I keep this oath faithfully, may I enjoy my life and practise my art, respected by all humanity and in all times; but if I swerve from it or violate it, may the reverse be my life."

Hypocratic Oath, Version 2, Wikipedia, January 2014

You can leave your hat on ...

A friend of mine tells a tall tale of a visit to a GP surgery. It was in the middle of winter and she was dressed in layer upon layer as she made her way to the surgery for a consultation over a niggling knee problem. She claims that when she finally made it into the doctor's room for her appointment, the doctor nonchalantly asked her to remove her clothes so that he could carry out a physical examination.

Somewhat surprised, my friend asked, "Do you mean that you want me to remove all my clothes? I've only come to see you about my knee."

"Well," the doctor retorted without even looking up from his notes. "You can leave your hat on."

This rather improbable account, though humorous, does however illustrate a serious point. We like to think that the training that doctors receive at university enables them to be unmoved by the sight of the naked human body and to view it with only pure academic interest. That way they can objectively assess disease without being distracted by prudish considerations. If this is true, I guess that makes doctors a bit superhuman in my view.

I am more inclined to believe that they are not, since many doctors I know are in normal relationships. As a result I am one of those people that remain somewhat uncomfortable about removing my clothes in front of doctors or nurses. I have no problem doing so in front of my partner but once I leave the secure confines of my house I do not look forward to removing my clothes for a stranger, even if that stranger is a doctor or nurse.

This probably sounds a bit silly and old-fashioned. After all, we all remove our clothes in front of strangers when lying on the beach. The difference though is that when we are on the beach there is virtually no chance of strangers touching us up the way doctors do when they are examining us. In addition, there is comfort in numbers. Somehow it's not so bad when there are thousands of you all in the same state of (un)dress.

I know doctors will protest at what I am saying. They don't really "touch us up". More often than not what they do is just gentle prodding, palpation using a couple of fingers or using a stethoscope or other instrument to check different organs. It is necessary, they rightly argue, for them to have some physical contact and to observe the uncovered body in order to make an accurate diagnosis.

I suppose I have to take doctors at their word when it comes to this. They in turn need to understand the trauma that some of their patients experience when being examined. It is said that a lot of patients experience the "white coat effect" when they see a doctor: their blood pressure rises at the sight of the doctor and gives a non-representative value.

I like to think that perhaps it's not just the sight of the coat that causes the blood pressure to rise. It's the fear of removing one's clothes and being probed all over.

The Appointment Game and My Local Surgery

Not too long ago I had that all-too-familiar sinking feeling when I realised I had no choice but to make an urgent appointment for my son at the surgery. As most of us know, doctors have a booking system that sometimes seems like it has been designed to dissuade you from trying to get an appointment.

The difficulty with making urgent appointment is that at my doctors' surgery, as in many other practices across the country, you can't call the day before and ask for an appointment with the doctor. You have to call at **8.30 am** and ask for any available slots that day. That sounds simple enough until you realise that there are tens or hundreds of other people all trying to do the same thing and you can't get through to the receptionist for 25 minutes. By the time you get through at about 9.00am; either all appointment slots are taken or you are asked to call again at about 11.30 am "when the doctor will be taking phone consultations."

74

I often wonder why nobody has attempted to solve this problem. Doctors up and down the country can't cope with the demand for their services and thus we have these solutions that are designed to create the illusion that patient's don't really have to wait more than a day for their appointments.

In classical economics "demand" currently far exceeds "supply". The textbook solution to the problem is to simply increase supply to meet demand at a more agreeable point. In other words, if the existing numbers of GPs are unable to cope with the requests from patients, the government should look at ways of training more GPs and easing the pressure. With my cynical hat on, I suspect that this has not happened because doctors have a very powerful union, the British Medical Association, and they (or someone in government) do not want the numbers of doctors to exceed a certain point relative to the population. A Daily Mail article lends credence to this theory by indicating that there are quotas on the numbers of students admitted onto medical courses every year as well as the numbers of doctors recruited. The risk, from the doctors' perspective, is that if there were more doctors, the "premium" on each doctor would decrease. Doctors would then earn less.

Whether or not you think that GP salaries are justified in view of the rigorous training they receive and the costs of education; my view on the availability of doctors is that numbers should be driven primarily by patient factors. The NHS exists for the benefit of patients. Doctors, pharmacists, nurses, dentists and other professionals employed by the NHS should have a patient-centred focus. This is currently not always the case. The urgent appointment system at GP surgeries is structured more for the convenience of GPs than the patients.

Let us, as patients, also get organised. We need to shift the power balance so that both GPs and the government start from the patients as a reference point, instead of the GP surgery. In the meantime, we are forced to keep playing the "find an appointment slot" game with GP surgeries.

The Irrational Patient

Sometimes as patients we argue as if everything we are saying is perfectly logical and bears equal weight to what the "experts" have to say. I am among those that have occasionally fallen into this trap.

Take, for instance, any time I develop unusual symptoms. The first thing I do before calling the doctor is to check on the internet what the symptoms indicate. More often than not I get a number of different diagnoses and then go for the one that I think most closely fits what I think are my symptoms; or what I suspect I might be getting; or any of various options. Usually by the time I get to the pharmacist or doctor I have convinced myself that I am suffering from the condition in mind and instead of giving a full list of symptoms for the professional to make a diagnosis I either hint or blatantly state what I think I'm suffering from.

I guess doctors and other health professionals must hate the internet for this. They spend years in university acquiring specialist training in order to be able to make accurate diagnoses and prescribe the right medication; only to be frustrated by patients that think that they are similarly qualified after spending a few hours on the internet. On behalf of those patients that realise the absurdity of this I wish to apologise to all hard-working, competent doctors and health professionals about this.

Of course the problem does not just relate to diagnosing illness. It extends to prescribing the treatment for illness as well. The media does not help matters when it comes to this. I have read on numerous occasions about so-called new "wonder drugs" that are much better than existing treatments. Often these are at the experimental and clinical trial stages; or they are being evaluated by the experts at NICE to see whether the evidence in favour of their use is solid. Yet, despite all this, we clamour for the drugs to be given to us or our loved ones on the basis that they reversed the symptoms in a number of people with symptoms similar to ours or those of our loved ones.

The difficulty with this stance is that it does not stand to proper scrutiny when weighed against best practice and history. The stories of Thalidomide and Vioxx® remind us of this fact. The truth is that when we are in situations in which we are trying to force doctors to prescribe specific drugs, we are acting out of desperation more than anything else. Often it is because existing treatments have failed to provide a cure and, in desperation, we clasp at straws as it were. We either wish to live, or we want our loved ones to live, so desperately that we are willing to take risks if there is any hope that there might be a favourable outcome. Doctors should understand our reasons for this.

A final example I give about our irrational choices is when it comes to placebos. I know I wrote about placebos a few chapters back – and how they should not be prescribed by ethical health professionals – but the truth is that all of us have at one time wanted one placebo or another.

Receptionists and Privacy

Ever had the urge to tell somebody − ever so politely − that the questions they were asking were really none of their business? I sometimes get that feeling when talking to some of the receptionists at my local surgery. Now, don't get me wrong. I appreciate the important role that receptionists play in organising the doctor's busy schedule and ensuring that all relevant correspondence relating to the treatment of patients gets to the attention of the doctor and is incorporated in the treatment records. I also appreciate that every important person has to have a personal assistant to act as a "gatekeeper" and filter out unnecessary intruders.

My problem is that some of the receptionists at my surgery are way too zealous in executing some of these functions; particularly the gatekeeping role. In a previous chapter I mourned about the difficulty of getting an appointment at my surgery. What I did not mention were the hoops and loops I have to jump through once I have made the connection. On an unlucky day the conversation can be something like this:

"Good morning. Doctor's surgery. Appointments. Can I help you?"

"Yes, please. My name is Pharma Patient, Date of Birth 01/01/1900. I'd like an appointment with one of the doctors today, please."

"What would you like the appointment for?"

"Pardon?"

"Why do you want to see the doctor? I need to see how urgent the request is."

"It's personal"

"But ...."

"I'd rather not discuss the issue with you, thank you. I prefer to talk to a proper doctor."

"Okay. We have an appointment at 10:50am with Doctor Who. Will that be okay?"

"Yes, that's fine. Thank you."

As I said above, it's not that I disrespect the role of the receptionist. I am also aware that they can probably see my medical records on their computer screens. However, as far as I know receptionists are not yet trained in evaluating a wide range of medical conditions or "triaging" patients according to the nature of the symptoms presented. I am not happy discussing my details with an unqualified person, no matter how well-intentioned. I also imagine that such interventions contribute to the lengthening of phone calls and the difficulties associated with getting through to the surgery in the first place.

The Ten-Minute Consultation

I first published this in October 2013 on my blog. I am led to believe that changes have now been incorporated into the GP contract so that from April 2014 it should be possible for patients to spend longer with their GPs at each consultation as well as have a greater choice in who could be their chosen GP in the first place. This should hopefully create a more "open" and fairer competitive environment resulting in measurable benefits for patients.

My original post was as follows:

"I went to see my GP today. It was over some tests for a long-term medical condition that needs to be monitored regularly.

I couldn't help noticing whilst in the waiting room that everybody seemed to spend only a few minutes with the GP for the consultation. I couldn't really tell if there was a difference between the amounts of time spent with male in contrast to female doctors. What I can say is that in the time that I was there, none of those in front of me in the queue spent more than ten minutes with any of the doctors at the practice.

This set me thinking: Logically doctors must ration the time that they spend with each patient in order to accommodate everyone that wants to be seen. The question is what the "gold standard" for a consultation is; and whether that is sufficient for the doctor to find out everything he/she needs to know about a patient and their medical conditions before prescribing treatment.

I decided to ask the pharmacist down the road. She indicated that she seemed to remember the consultation period being usually around ten minutes somewhere in the doctors' contract; but since she wasn't a doctor herself she wouldn't want to commit herself to that figure. When I got home I decided to look it up and came across the following from the British Medical Journal careers website:

"Now, most GPs offer 10 minutes for routine appointments, which is recognised in the GP contract as an indicator of quality. But 10 minutes may not be enough, given that GPs are increasingly dealing with chronic and complex conditions, a growing elderly population, health promotion targets, and the need to bring care closer to home."

On the one hand it is reassuring to learn that GPs themselves are aware that sometimes the consultation time is just not long enough and they are talking about extending it where warranted. On the other it makes me worry that I might have been prescribed inappropriate or inadequate treatment in the past because my GP did not take enough time to listen to me or check my symptoms.

Could I have been exposed to unnecessary side effects or made to suffer unnecessarily longer, I wonder?"

Patients and Placebos

I cannot speak for all patients, but I admit that I have contradictory views about placebos. In an earlier chapter I berated pharmacists for selling placebos in the form of homeopathic medicines. This was a tad hypocritical because, in most cases, I accept the word of a health professional as fact and will do what my doctor or pharmacist tells me to do.

For instance, if a doctor or pharmacist recommends a cough mixture for a troublesome cough, I take their word and get the prescribed medicine. I try it out for a week or so and then go back if it hasn't worked. In the case of a cough it is probably debatable whether any improvements are due to the medicine or not. Most coughs will resolve naturally within a period of one to three weeks. However, expediency tends to override academic debate in these situations. Any form of treatment seems better than none.

The same view holds for me in any other desperate position. I am not alone in this. One of my friends tried a number of over-the-counter and prescribed medicines for an unexplained hip problem. None of them wears effective.

In the end one of the doctors at her surgery suggested acupuncture but provided a healthy dose of scepticism on the effectiveness of the technique since it does not seem to make sense from a western medical viewpoint. This did not deter her and she actually found acupuncture more effective than any of the drugs she had tried up to that point.

There are two other reasons I find that I am willing to accept placebos in my treatment even though I know that they are not effective from a strictly scientific perspective. Firstly, I am not willing to discount the power of the placebo effect. Even the best double-blind, placebo controlled clinical trials assume that there will be a beneficial effect associated with the use of a placebo. In fact, the odds of getting some benefit from a placebo are much greater than some of the other risks we regard as acceptable. It is generally accepted that the placebo effect will account for anything from ten to fifty percent of perceived benefits of a treatment, with thirty percent accepted as an average figure. Compare that with the odds associated with betting on a horse or the lottery and suddenly a placebo appears much more reasonable.

Associated with the probability considerations is the fact that there are aspects of the placebo effect that are difficult to explain. I am told, for instance, that some animals have been shown to benefit from homeopathic medicines. I do not know how good the studies that claimed to show this effect were but, if true, it certainly calls for some explaining. Besides this, people of various faiths will often cite miraculous healing that does not fit the realm of science as we know it. It is probably stretching it a bit to equate such healing with the placebo effect but I mention the two together since the recipient's outlook is a key element of the effectiveness of both faith healing and the placebo effect.

The final reason I am willing to consider placebos is that I do not have the training or inclination to assess every possible treatment I receive from my health professional. There is a certain level of competence and training required to evaluate, understand and form an accurate understanding of all the trials that relate to the treatment of medical conditions. Health professionals spend years training hour to do this and we have organisations such as NICE and the MHRA whose duty it is to evaluate treatments before recommending them to health professionals as suitable for patients. I think it would be naïve of me to assume that a few hours spent on Google would suffice for me to have a balanced and accurate view about a treatment. If a doctor decided to give me an injection of water for my complaint, I would probably accept it without further questions.

What does this mean for doctors? I am not suggesting that doctors start prescribing and giving placebos. This is probably a bad idea due to the non-predictability of the placebo effect. I am merely suggesting that perhaps doctors and other health professionals could leverage the placebo effect in regular treatments. If, for instance, it is more likely that I will take a medicine and benefit because of the recommendation of a health professional, the doctor and pharmacist could spend a few extra seconds highlighting the benefits of complying with treatment. If an elderly patient prefers an injection to oral medication, giving her that antibiotic via injection might be more beneficial than expecting her to take a course of large, difficult-to-swallow capsules for a week or two.

You get the idea, I think …

Training Days

Doctors' practices are meant to exist for the benefit of patients. Sometimes I wonder if the opposite is true. Take for example one Wednesday in January 2014 when I tried to call my surgery for some urgent advice possibly leading to an appointment. This was a regular Wednesday and not a bank holiday.

I got an unpleasant surprise when the message on the answer phone indicated that the surgery was "shut for training". It was evident that there were no doctors available to attend to patients and that the receptionists would not answer the phone. In panic I called the pharmacy to find out what was happening and to check my options. They explained that the receptionists had informed them that morning that they would be shut in the afternoon as all the doctors had to attend some special training. Although the receptionists were on the premises undertaking other administrative work, the surgery would not be open to patients for routine appointments. Patients had the option of calling NHS Direct, going to the pharmacy, Walk-in Centre or even A & E.

I was shocked and disappointed. I did not expect to have to go to these lengths to access treatment that should normally be readily accessible at my surgery. I quickly checked the surgery website and found that it had not been updated with the details of the closure. I had been to the surgery a few days before and did not recall seeing a notice that the surgery would be shut a few days thence. I thought that the failure to notify patients in good time smacked of arrogance.

I was also not convinced that it had been absolutely necessary to close the surgery. As far as I know there are locum GPs available that could have been called upon to provide essential care if it was necessary for all the regular GPs to attend a training session. There are whole practices that seem to operate on locums. Why my surgery felt this was beyond them I have no clue.

I know that pharmacies have a contractual obligation to remain open a certain number of hours per week as indicated under the terms of their contract with the NHS. When they fail to do so they can face fines or more severe penalties, including the withdrawal of their contracts for persistent offenders. I am not sure if there is a similar system in place for doctors' surgeries.

On the positive side such instances rarely happen at my local surgery. The problem is that when they do, there can be serious consequences for patients. My request to all GPs therefore is that they avoid such instances at all costs. If they are unavoidable, at least they should make an effort to notify patients well in advance. Common courtesy demands this.

GP Influence and the NHS

This chapter shares my thoughts on the influence of GPs within the NHS. This stems from an observation that GPs, over the past ten years or so, appear to be gaining a stronger influence on the NHS than they have in previous periods. You can get a very good history of the NHS on the website of the Nuffield Trust.

Contractor GPs appear to have got a very good deal in the changes to the GP contract in 2003-04, with a lot experiencing around a sixty percent increase in their earnings. Some of them managed to get much higher increases. This was despite the fact that the new contract allowed GPs to effectively reduce their working hours and to be shut on weekends. It introduced a number of elements such as practice-based commissioning and the quantitative outcomes framework.

If the major broadsheets are to be believed, full-time GPs were earning around £55,000 to £65,000 per annum in 2004. This jumped to between £105,000 and £120,000 after the changes to the contract. Some were said to be earning much higher than this – in the region of £300,000 and greater. Of course the response from some of the GPs has been that they were underpaid before the new contract was introduced. Those with long memories will remember how the 2012 GP strikes brought the question of GP pay into focus. This period possibly marked the lowest ebb in the popularity of the doctors.

Why do I mention the changes in GP remuneration? It seems odd that only GPs have experienced such massive improvements in their earnings at a time when the NHS has had to make cost savings in other areas. I am led to understand that not long afterwards a new contract was introduced for pharmacists but it did not bring such massive increments. This is despite the fact that pharmacists (like nurses) are now undertaking roles that used to be associated purely with doctors. My local pharmacist spends time talking to me about my use of my medicines. In fact, I usually get more time with the pharmacist than with the doctor. When I visit the surgery, I often see a nurse prescriber instead of the doctor. I have even been surprised to consult with pharmacist prescribers. My pharmacist also provides many more services than she did ten years ago.

I have not investigated the dentist contract at any length; hence it is difficult to say whether dentists are better off or worse off than in the past. What I do know is that it is still not easy to get an appointment with an NHS dentist. On the other hand, if you want private treatment the service is considerably faster.

In 2013 further changes were introduced to the NHS. These saw eighty billion pounds of NHS funds channelled through clinical commissioning groups that were mainly led by GPs. Primary care trusts and local health boards were abolished among other changes. As we are in the first year of these changes at the time of writing this chapter, we are still to see how beneficial the new structure is in comparison with the previous arrangements.

Notable in all this however is the assumption by politicians that "doctors know best." Perhaps this follows from the fact that the health minister is a doctor himself. However, from the choice descriptions given of the minister by doctors in online forums, I get the impressions that he is not popular among his fellow professionals either.

I think politicians miss out by not conferring more with other health professionals. Nurses nowadays are trained to degree level and can specialise in several disciplines. They are arguably the mainstay of community-based healthcare for vulnerable groups. Most well-run GP surgeries work hand-in-hand with community nurses with this in mind. As indicated above, even within surgeries there are often nurse prescribers that take a considerable burden off the shoulders of GPs.

Pharmacists are similarly not given adequate attention. In hospital settings they play a crucial role in checking dosages in wards. In the community they perform a range of functions from the traditional dispensing role to checking all sorts of prescriptions, providing a range of services and even prescribing. In fact, discussions with my pharmacist friends reveal that since around 2001 pharmacists have graduated with a Masters level degree from all universities in the UK.

In practice the average community nurse, pharmacist and GP provide an integrated service with seamless care of patients, yet the respective contracts for these professions are still based on the premise that the professions are virtually working in independent silos save for some forced areas of collaboration.

We need some more joined-up thinking on the part of those that draw the contracts for GPs, pharmacists and services such as those provided by community nurses. This would require that other health professions be involved in the setting up of the frameworks for contracts with GPs, and vice versa, so that clear synergies and areas of collaboration can be identified. The current system in which pharmacists (or dentists) await the conclusion of the GP contract before commencing their own negotiations perpetuates the perception that the primary care component of the NHS is mainly about GPs, with pharmacists, community nurses, dentists and other health care providers scrambling for the leftover pieces.

Section 3: Other Parts of Primary Care

"We are clear that Government cannot – and should not – pretend it can 'make' the population healthy. But it can – and should – support people in making better choices for their health."

Prime Minister Tony Blair, in Department of Health (2004) *Choosing Health: Making healthy choices easier.* Department of Health.

"NHS Direct is here to make a difference to the lives of people in England. 24-hours a day, 365 days a year."

What is NHS Direct? www.nhsdirect.nhs.uk, 1998.

Source: *Nuffield Trust.* http://nhstimeline.nuffieldtrust.org.uk/

NHS Direct

NHS Direct is a relatively recent addition to the National Health Service, having been introduced in 1998. In the first few years of its existence I was among the many millions that called the old number 0845 46 47 for advice about a number of health issues. This was before I had access to the internet.

The phone service was, in my view, excellent. I could not believe it when I found out through a friend that the people at the other end of the line were not necessarily fully qualified health professionals; but well-trained staff that followed a computer algorithm on how to handle a range of common queries. Their ability to evaluate various situations and come up with an appropriate recommendation was impressive. I fully expect that they made a number of mistakes but my impression of them overall was very positive.

Later on as I got a reliable broadband internet connection at home I ventured onto the NHS Direct website. It proved to be very well-designed and a useful reference source that I still use to this day. What I like about the website is its simplicity and the fact that it is very intuitive to use. On the home page you are given the option to check your own symptoms, find out about health conditions, keep healthy in all seasons or find your nearest health services (GP, pharmacy, dentist or A&E department). What I especially like about the website is that it is not cluttered with Google advertisements like many of the other health websites that I sometimes visit. This perhaps adds more credence to the site in that it is not commercially driven but is focused purely on providing impartial health information.

Overall I cannot fault the NHS Direct service. It fits well the rest of the NHS family and stands head and shoulders with the best health resources around.

Walk-In Centres

As far as I can recall I have had to use Walk-In Centres on four occasions in my life. One of these was for a personal problem whereas the other three related to family members. I am as pleased with the experience at the Walk-In Centres as I am with NHS Direct.

The experience is simple enough. You go to the centre with a medical problem; a nurse assesses how urgent your need is; you wait in line and somebody else examines you before deciding whether to give you any treatment or refer you further. The nurses prescribe any medication that you need and there is often a pharmacy nearby to dispense any required medication.

In the main I found that the nurses that I encountered at the Centres still had the caring side to their nature despite the challenges that they face. It must be difficult to maintain an operation that is open twelve hours a day throughout the year and still maintain a cheerful outlook all the time. My hat goes off to the nurses that work at these places.

PHARMAPATIENT'S LIFE AT THE RECEIVING END

I also commend the politicians that came up with the idea to have such places. These are some of the things that make the NHS great.

Dentist Services

Giving an opinion about NHS dental services is difficult for me. The reason for this is simple: I do not have recent experience of using them and thus cannot give a true evaluation of them. This might appear unusual to some people but there is a strong underlying cause.

Several years ago my partner and I moved to a new city for work. After registering with a local GP we tried to find an NHS dentist as well. This was not easy but we eventually found one. When we called up to make an appointment for registration we were told that we would have to make an initial appearance for the first check before registration could be confirmed. The only problem was that the earliest appointment was more than three months from that date.

Meanwhile there was an option for us to join a private dental health scheme through my partner's employee benefits. This guaranteed speedy access to a dentist and good quality care at a moderate cost. Rather than wait for the NHS dentist we opted to go private. I cannot remember if our current dentist (whom we see privately) is the one that we had tried to register with via the NHS.

I hope my experience was not the norm. It would be sad if essential and urgent patient care were regularly delayed because of lengthy waits for appointments at dental surgeries. This suggests that the government needs to divert more funds to train dentists and allow more practices to open so as to improve accessibility.

The Complex National Health Service

As a patient it is easy to take the National Health Service for granted. Most of the people that will read this short book will have lived all their lives with the guarantee of the NHS or equivalent health systems in other countries. I hope I have presented both the good and the bad sides of the primary care end of the system.

I think GPs, community nurses and pharmacists do a wonderful job. Sometimes things go wrong and it is natural to mourn about these but in the main most people realize that they are relatively lucky in this country. You only need to go on holiday abroad and need medical care to realize what it means to have the NHS back home.

I have not covered the care provided by hospitals as that is a bit sensitive at the moment in light of the Stafford Hospital Scandal that has been in the media for the past few years. Perhaps I will try to look at hospitals in a future book.

I also thought of writing about the way in which the government has tinkered with the structure of the NHS despite – according to some - there not being a strong enough case for the changes. When I looked at the history of the NHS, however, I saw that the structure undergoes changes every few years. I am not sure how long the current incarnation of the system will last. It is possible that the election of a new party into government would lead to another reorganisation. I suppose the best approach is to allow each version enough time to prove itself before passing judgment.

With such a wonderful service there is always the potential for abuse. As a patient I get really upset when I read stories of how people defraud and abuse the system. There are those who are working but fail to pay their fair share of the comparatively small NHS levy. It is only a token fee in comparison with the true cost of treatment. Then there are those who choose to find ways of fleecing the system as private contractors providing services and goods either to or on behalf of the system. Some of these are health professionals that claim for services or products that they have not provided. The problem with all this is that it reduces the funds available to the genuinely ill that need treatment. I am not even going to start on the health tourists that visit the country to get treatment and then flee without paying for it …

Finally, I sometimes wonder how long we'll have the NHS for. We are constantly being reminded how the NHS does not have infinite capacity for dealing with the nation's ills; how the ageing population is a potential time bomb as we will not have adequate resources in future to deal with the demands on the system; and how we cannot afford new and more expensive but more effective drugs. I personally think it all boils down to priorities. There are personal decisions that we as patients have to make: decisions on lifestyle that determine how likely we are to fall sick and suffer from the common lifestyle diseases related to poor dietary and lifestyle choices. As a country there are also big decisions that we need to make on how national finances are spent.

Perhaps the NHS needs to shift from a treatment to a preventative focus; gently nudging people towards making more healthy lifestyle choices. In an ideal world I would like to think this is possible. In the real world of cheap and fast junk food, booze promotions, easy availability of tobacco and general glamorization of "living for the moment", however, I doubt we'll see a realization of this ideal any time soon.

Concluding Remarks: How to Make Your Patients Happy

As a parting shot I thought I would add ten personal suggestions for health professionals on how to have a happy clientele. As with everything else these are the humble suggestions of one patient among millions that rely on the NHS. They might prove useful in future if you give them a bit of thought.

1. **When you are attending to me, make me feel like I'm the most important thing to you at that moment**. Most patients just want to be heard, to have the assurance that their concerns are taken seriously and to know that everything possible is being done to address the concerns.

2. **Make me feel that I can trust you**. Most patients confide some very personal things to their health professional. It is almost as if the consultation room is a sacred space. Violate this trust at your peril. This also includes not using me as a guinea pig without my consent.

3. **Do not misuse anything about me**. In the modern world of Twitter®, Facebook® and other easy forms of publicizing information, do not feel like you have the liberty to tell the world things about me. If I find out that you like making fun of your patients, I am not likely to want to see you about any of my health problems. If I find myself the butt of your jokes online, expect to hear from my lawyer.

4. **Give me enough time**. I know you have to ration your time among a thousand people per day but when I have problem you need to spend enough time with me to properly understand what my problem is and how you can treat it. "A stitch in time saves nine," so the old saying goes. If you take the right amount of time to understand and treat me the first time, it can save us both a lot of time in future.

5. **Treat me like a human being**. I know you have targets of one sort or another and get paid by how many of those targets you have hit. For GPs I know that you get so many QOF points for recording things about patients, whereas in pharmacy it can be about getting that extra MUR or getting more items to hit your target. Stop thinking about me and my

prescription or conditions in terms of statistics. I am a human being with feelings, fears and emotions. I am normally driven to see you by the pain and discomfort of the underlying illness; coupled with fear. It might be fear of death or the fear of what could happen to my loved ones if something happened to me. I need you to understand this. When you do, you will treat me more like a person than just another number.

6. **If you can't help, be honest and tell me**. Some people are too proud to admit when they don't know or cannot help. Since we are dealing with my life here, I would rather you tell me straightaway when you don't know than pretend to know and experiment on me without my knowledge. I know you can sometimes be lucky and chance on the right treatment, but I do not want to be the unlucky person for whom a delay in treatment results in illness progressing to a stage where it is no longer treatable. If you let me know early on, at least I have a greater chance of finding treatment from someone who knows.

7. **Do not abuse me**. This is different to number 3 above. Sometimes I am in a position in which I stand in awe of you as a health professional. There is an imbalance of power between us, no matter how you look at it. You hold more power than I do. This places a huge responsibility on you to maintain a professional distance and not take advantage of that. Having an affair with me is certainly verging onto forbidden ground. Just ask yourself, before you do anything to/with me, if it would stand the scrutiny of your fellow peers in an unbiased public panel.

8. **Respect my wishes**. I know I am not a qualified health professional but I have some personal preferences that are driven by factors I regard as greater than accepted logic or science. This means that sometimes I will listen to what you have to say and still do the complete opposite. This might be because of my views and fears that transcend facts and figures. Please respect my right to hold opinions that are stronger than your arguments on anything from abortion to the right to terminate one's life in cases of terminal illness.

9. **Do not lie to me**. I prefer that you tell me about my condition and treatments as fully and simply as possible. This includes information on the risks or the relative benefits of treatment. Sometimes you may be tempted to hide the truth under big words so that you do not have to explain in detail; whereas at other times you might feel that you have to push a particular treatment that you do not believe is effective. Allow me the chance to make an informed based on a balance of objective information. I guess this also places a responsibility on you to ensure that any information that you bring to my attention has been thoroughly vetted for reliability. The case of the MMR scandal comes to mind.

10. **Bo not treat me differently because of my social standing**. I know there is a temptation to treat the rich and famous in a manner that differs from the poor and lowly. However, a less privileged background is no reason for me to get substandard care. I may have disheveled hair, not have had a decent bath and change of clothes in a while, or be sleeping rough; but your non-judgmental treatment might be the only ray of light I see in an otherwise gloomy world. In any case, the world has a funny

way of turning things round: one minute I could be down in the dumps; the next I could be a millionaire.

About the Author

Pharmapatient is an anonymous patient using the National Health Service in England. Not much is known about Pharmapatient other than the few glimpses seen through this book: a partner, some children and the frequenting of GP practices and pharmacies. It is the last of these that forms the basis for the stories and opinions expressed in the book.

The author takes us on a journey that flows through frustration at being seen as just another medical statistic, the profundity of the life-saving work provided by health professionals and the consideration of how efficiently different parts of the National Health Service are run. The insights gained should prove revealing to both patients and health professionals alike.

CPSIA information can be obtained at www.ICGtesting.com
Printed in the USA
LVOW10s1819020315

428941LV00001B/137/P